MW00962645

Ketogenic Diet

Lose Up to 20 Pounds, 4 Inches-
-and Restore Overall Health!—
in 21 Days

Andrew Manson

© **Copyright 2016 by Andrew Manson - All rights reserved.**

This document is geared towards providing exact and reliable information in regards to the topic and issue covered. The publication is sold with the idea that the publisher is not required to render accounting, officially permitted, or otherwise, qualified services. If advice is necessary, legal or professional, a practiced individual in the profession should be ordered.

- From a Declaration of Principles which was accepted and approved equally by a Committee of the American Bar Association and a Committee of Publishers and Associations.

In no way is it legal to reproduce, duplicate, or transmit any part of this document in either electronic means or in printed format. Recording of this publication is strictly prohibited and any storage of this document is not allowed unless with written permission from the publisher. All rights reserved.

The information provided herein is stated to be truthful and consistent, in that any liability, in terms of inattention or otherwise, by any usage or abuse of any policies, processes, or directions contained within is the solitary and utter responsibility of the recipient reader. Under no circumstances will any legal responsibility or blame be held against the publisher for any reparation, damages, or monetary loss due to the information herein, either directly or indirectly.

Respective authors own all copyrights not held by the publisher.

The information herein is offered for informational purposes solely, and is universal as so. The presentation of the information is without contract or any type of guarantee assurance.

The trademarks that are used are without any consent, and the publication of the trademark is without permission or backing by the trademark owner. All trademarks and brands within this book are for clarifying purposes only and are the owned by the owners themselves, not affiliated with this document.

Table of Contents

Introduction

I would like to thank you for downloading the book, *"Ketogenic Diet: Lose Up to 20 Pounds, 4 Inches--and Restore Overall Health!—in Just 21 Days (Includes 30 Fat Destroying Recipes, 21-Day Diet Meal Plan, and 10 Tips for Success)."*

Currently, obesity and other metabolic diseases have proved to be the world's greatest health challenge. According to statistics, more than 2.8 million obesity-related deaths are recorded among adults each year. Other reports show that metabolic syndrome affects at least 50 million people in the United States and often triggers various health problems.

To deal with these emerging issues, many diet plans have been formulated but only a few of them are scientifically proven. One of the most efficient diets recommended in managing obesity and related diseases is Ketogenic diet. Are you wondering what the ketogenic diet is and how it can help you lose weight, be healthier and live a longer fulfilling life? Wonder no more, because this book has everything you need to know about the ketogenic diet.

Designed as the ultimate Ketogenic Diet Guide, this book will help you know more about the ketogenic diet; what it is, benefits of going on the diet, how to lose weight while on the diet and so much more.

Thanks again for downloading this book. I hope you enjoy it!

Chapter 1:
Understanding The Ketogenic Diet

The Ketogenic diet is basically a low carb, high fat, moderate protein diet. The term Ketogenic is derived from "Keto" which means "ketone" and "genic" which means to produce. In order to understand the ketogenic diet, it is critical to understand the science behind this diet.

The Science Behind The Keto Diet

Basically, the body has a preference for glucose as a source of energy. Thus, when you take a diet high in carbohydrates, the body breaks down the carbohydrates into glucose and the body uses the glucose for energy. Normally insulin hormone is produced to manage blood glucose levels; thus, insulin enables the cells to use the glucose and initiates the process of dealing with any excess glucose. Excess glucose is converted to glycogen and stored in the liver and muscles and any remaining excess is converted into fatty acids and stored in adipose tissue.

When on a low carb diet, the body does not have ready glucose available for energy; hence, it has to look for other sources of energy. The body begins by breaking down the glycogen into glucose. Since this is not enough to meet the body's demand for energy, the liver breaks down the fatty acids into ketones, which the body uses for energy.

As you have read, the ketogenic diet is very effective at burning any excess fat stored and thus it is very effective for weight loss. But how much carbohydrates, proteins and fat should you eat in order to initiate the ketosis process (breaking down of fatty acids into ketones).

How To Initiate Ketosis

To trigger ketosis, you should restrict carb intake to 50 grams per day, which means that only 5-10 percent of calories should be from carbs. Also eat a high fat diet comprising of 70-75 percent of fat and 20-25 percent of proteins.

But why eat more fats? For starters, fat has no significant effect on blood sugar levels and thus no great effect on insulin, which initiates conversion of excess glucose into fat. In addition, fat will provide you with the energy you need.

It is also important to moderate your protein intake as protein can affect blood sugar and insulin levels too. Actually, any extra protein is converted into glucose in what is called *gluconeogenesis* and this affects blood sugar and insulin levels. As rise in insulin facilitates glucose metabolism, this hinders ketone production and overall fat loss.

To avoid conversion of protein to glucose, limit intake to about 1-1.5 grams per each kilo of lean body mass. An optimum intake of protein and extremely low carb diet facilitate oxidation of stored body fats into ketones, a process called *ketosis*.

With that in mind, where did the Keto diet originate from? Here's a brief history of the diet plan:

The History Of The Ketogenic Diet

The diet was designed in 1920s by Dr. Henry Rawle Geyelin, an endocrinologist determined to treat drug-resistant epilepsy. The doctor realized that fasting changed the way the body processed nutrients and this helped reduce seizures in patients.

In his studies, Geyelin found out that during fasting, glucose concentration in the blood reduced while the level of ketones increased. While the body metabolized ketones for fuel rather than glucose, the likelihood of seizures occurring was greatly reduced.

Geyelin opted to maintain high production of ketones for longer periods of time which lead to formulation of the Ketogenic diet. His initial Keto diet was mainly dedicated to treating epileptic children in 1930's until *anticonvulsant* medications were introduced.

Later in 1994, the Keto diet became famous again after Jim Abrahams, a Hollywood producer adopted it to treat his epileptic child. Then, Charlie Abrahams, an epileptic victim, greatly reduced seizure occurrence from a hundred daily to no-seizure at all drug-free. A further promotion by Charlie Foundation through movies and news reports saw the diet widely accepted as form of therapy.

So far, studies have shown that the Keto diet can reduce occurrence of seizures by more than half. As the diet becomes more popular, many people have successfully applied it for other reasons such as weight loss.

In the following chapter, we are going to look at benefits of adopting the ketogenic diet other than weight loss.

Chapter 2:
Living Healthier And Longer With The Keto Diet

Since the invention of Agriculture, our diet has drastically changed. Compared to the Ancient Man or the Hunter Gatherers, intake of protein has reduced by about 10-15 percent while carb intake increased by 45-60 percent! A more disturbing fact is that we're now over-indulging on grains and starch products rather than nutritious fruits and veggies. The carbs we eat have high glycemic load or glycemic index which our bodies aren't fully adopted to metabolize. Such a diet is a big challenge and a source of stress for our bodies.

Worse still, intake of unsaturated fats from foods like fish has greatly reduced with a sharp increase in saturated fats. Poly-unsaturated and mono-unsaturated fats are healthy for the brain and heart function. Our diets are instead comprised of more processed fats such as Trans fatty acids. According to research, unhealthy fats are linked to cardiovascular problems, high cholesterol and other metabolic disorders.

But with Keto diet, carb intake is drastically reduced and you now focus on healthier fats for weight loss and optimal health. That being said, here are the benefits of Keto diet:

Health Benefits Of The Keto Diet

Adopting the ketogenic diet can lead to a number of benefits including:

Weight and Fat Loss

The Keto diet can both help you burn fat and lose weight within a few weeks. Research has shown that when equal number of calories are consumed across different diet plans, a low-carb diet facilitates a greater extent of fat loss.

In a study, scientists compared three different meal plans that contained varying amounts of carbs i.e. 104, 60 and 30 grams of carbs. They discovered a negative correlation between carbs consumed and weight loss. Low carb diet (30 grams) proved to be more effective in both losing weight and conserving muscle mass.

Another research found out that when around 10 grams of carbs was consumed for 10 days, participants were able to lose 97 percent of their total body fat. Actually, a low carb diet is very effective even in obese people and doesn't require dieters to restrict intake of calories to lose fat. Further, a study observed that eating high amounts of fats and proteins is more effective in weight loss compared to low-fat diet.

Long term, and past 1 year studies have shown that a Keto diet is more effective for weight loss than conventional diets for the first 6 months. Therefore, with strong will power to achieve proper adherence to Keto diet, you can actually lose more weight when on a ketogenic diet

Curbs Hunger

The Ketogenic diet also promotes satiety or fullness. Thus, this will avoid unnecessary cravings that cause you to snack on processed or high-carb foods. In a particular study, one group of obese dieters were put on 30 percent protein diet and 4 percent carbs while the other group fed on 35 percent carbs. Then their body weight and level of ketosis was evaluated using their urine samples and analysis of blood plasma. A computerized system was used to assess and analyze their hunger patterns within a 4 week period.

After the 4 weeks, dieters who consumed 4 percent carb diet had a lower consumption of energy and reduced hunger than those who ate 35 percent of carbs. This study concluded that eating a low-carb and moderate protein Keto diet can help reduce hunger and food intake on short-term basis.

A related research found out that obese and non-diabetic overweight dieters can effectively reduce their appetite and lose 13 percent of body weight while on the ketogenic diet.

Other benefits of adopting the ketogenic diet is improved insulin sensitivity, reduced risk of cardiovascular problems, reduced risk of suffering from high blood pressure, long life among others.

If you want to lose weight fast with the Keto diet, the following chapter will focus on how you can get started and maintain the dieting plan.

Chapter 3:
Getting Started On The Keto Diet

Adapting a new diet or eating lifestyle can be challenging especially for a beginner. Another challenge is that the modern diet is high in processed foods and carbohydrates; thus, adopting a healthy low carb diet can be challenging because high carb processed foods seem to be everywhere.

In order to adopt the Ketogenic diet successfully, you need to prepare adequately; you need a specific strategy to make both your body and brain adapt. Thus, let us learn how you can do this.

Planning Your Diet

Doing a simple meal plan in advance can help you gather required supplies and avoid unnecessary time wastage. Though this might seem difficult or complicated at first, the basics involves getting rid of foods you should not eat from your kitchen, stocking your kitchen with the accepted foods, deciding your recipes, grouping the ingredients based on their preparation time and preparing those requiring more time in advance.

You can also deal with ingredients that require separate preparation and later assemble everything together. For instance, it saves time to soak the nuts, or prepare the nut cheese and pesto in advance before you make the breakfast or dessert pizza. You can also make chocolate drizzle in advance to later incorporate into various chocolate recipes and save considerable amount of time.

If you find your new meal plan hard to implement, begin with those simple meals that require locally available ingredients from supermarkets, groceries or local markets. Replace one meal every day with a low carb meal until you can successfully go on a low carb diet. To start you off, here are guidelines that can make the transition as effortless as possible:

Tips For Success

1. Get rid of keto unfriendly foods because this will make the process easier. We will look at foods to eat and those to avoid in a later chapter.

2. Ensure that you buy enough supply of fresh whole foods, fruits and veggies; then gradually expand your pantry with Keto friendly foodstuffs.

3. Make substitutes for processed foods. For instance, while you should avoid store bought ice cream because it is high in carbohydrates and sugar, you can instead make homemade ice cream with healthier alternatives. Also, instead of having your usual white flour pancakes, you can instead make almond pancakes, which are not as high in carbohydrates.

4. Buy organic products from credible sources to avoid those chemicals used in most conventional crops

5. Add fresh herbs, spices and seasonings to various recipes as flavors make most foods delicious, while herbs promote health and fight diseases.

6. Drink at least 8 cups of water daily as staying hydrated helps in flushing out toxins from the body, and can also help fight occasional cravings.

7. Adopt an active lifestyle as exercising helps boost your brain power, burn calories, build muscle and fight lifestyle diseases.. Try walking, jogging, swimming, yoga or other cardio-vascular activity.

8. Get enough vitamins as they support weight loss by strengthening your body cells, muscles, and bones. Most fruits and veggies are rich in vitamin A, B, C and K as well as other phytonutrients.

9. Manage your stress levels because when you are stressed, the stress hormones elevate blood sugar levels and this can interfere with ketosis especially when you are stressed for a long time.

10. Have adequate sleep because it is really challenging to stick to any diet when you are not well rested and have the ability to make the best decisions.

That said; it's normal to face challenges here and there but being aware of possible pitfalls can make recovery easier. Here are 3 common mistakes and how to avoid them:

Keto Diet Mistakes To Avoid

1. Failure to monitor your blood sugar levels

While the Ketogenic diet helps lower insulin levels and boost sugar tolerance, be aware that chronic carb starvation or absence of insulin hormone can hinder leptin release. Leptin detects hunger and its absence may discourage eating or slow-down metabolism. Therefore, as much as you want relatively stable blood sugar levels, you don't want to suffer from hypoglycemia.

2. Not eating enough foods high in fiber

Dietary fiber doesn't raise your blood sugar level as carbs do but instead makes you feel fuller for longer and fights cravings. Fiber works by slowing down glucose absorption in the blood, which avoids unnecessary sugar spikes that can trigger insulin production. Therefore, get plenty of fiber from whole unprocessed foods such as leafy green veggies and fresh fruits.

3. Eating Less Fat

Keto diet is low in carb so you need to substitute with high energy foods such as fats and proteins. A lower fat intake lowers your calorie intake, which slows down production of energy and you're thus unable to sustain a Keto diet. Simply ensure 60-75 percent of calories you eat come from healthy fatty foods and oils.

As stated before, you also need to limit intake of carbs to 50 grams and proteins as any excess will be converted to glucose. To follow the diet as it should be, you must learn the foods to put onto your plate and how to eat them in 21 days. Let's discuss that next:

Chapter 4: Eating On The Keto Diet

As already stated, the bulk of the Ketogenic diet is fats and oils as well as moderate protein intake. These have to be taken in the right proportion as stated before to achieve the benefits of a Ketogenic diet. Let's see which foods you should embrace:

What Your Plate Should Have

1. Fats and Oils

The most recommended fats to eat are omega 3 fatty oils, from sources such as fish like salmon, tuna and trout just to mention a few. Additionally, take saturated and mono saturated fats from butter, macadamia nuts, avocados, egg yolks and coconut oils. These fats are preferred because they have a stable chemical structure, which is less inflammatory.

2. Protein

This food group forms a considerable part of the Ketogenic diet plan as it facilitates general growth as well as repair of worn out cells. Protein also help in the synthesis and monitoring of hormones in the blood stream that control various bodily functions. Eat protein from sources such as fish like catfish, salmon, trout, tuna, mackerel and cod fish. You can also eat chicken, duck, turkey, pork, goats lamb and cattle.

3. Veggies

These are sources of vitamins that enhance your immune system to fight diseases, especially the leafy green veggies. However, veggies allowed in Keto diet should be high in nutrients and low in carbohydrates, thus avoid starchy carbs.

Eat leafy green veggies such as kales, cucumber, broccoli, asparagus, collard greens and mushrooms among others.

Apart from these food groups, you can also eat moderate amounts of fruits, nuts, seeds and spices.

Before we get to the Keto recipes you can try, here a simple shopping guide that you can follow:

Your Keto Diet Shopping Guide

Fruits and Veggies

Bell peppers
Onion
Tomatoes
Yellow squash
Flat-leaf parsley
Mushrooms
Spinach
Romaine lettuce
Zucchini
Jalapeno pepper
Cauliflower
Eggplant
Parsley flakes
Carrots
Radishes
Kale
Cucumbers
Cabbage
Artichoke hearts
Broccoli
Asparagus
Bok Choy
Berries
Avocado

Meat, Fish, Eggs and Poultry
Eggs
Bacon
Chorizo
Chicken breasts/sticks
Lobster
Haddock
Scallops
Deveined shrimp
Ham
Pork sausage rinds
Ground turkey
Italian sausage
Duck's breast
Turkey pepperoni
Lean deli ham
Canned tuna

Dairy, Fats and Oils
Olive oil
Butter
Cheddar/ Roquefort
/Jack/Swiss/Mozzarella/Parmesan/Cream/Cottage cheese
Milk
Heavy whipping cream
Cooking spray
Sour cream
Vegetable oil
Organic coconut oil
Evaporated milk

Nuts and Seeds
Pecans
Celery seed
Sesame seeds
Tahini
Walnuts
Almond
Flax seed
Sunflower seeds

Spices and sweeteners
Ground cumin
Garlic cloves and garlic powder
Paprika
Salt
Pepper
Marinara sauce
Vanilla extract
Oregano
Splenda
Ground cinnamon
Hot sauce
Red wine
Balsamic vinegar
Mustard
Hot chili pepper
Soy sauce
Dry sherry
Cayenne pepper
Nutmeg
Sweet basil/basil leaves
Tomato sauce
Ground white/black pepper
Dried thyme leaves

Hot pepper sauce
Rosemary
Italian seasoning
Orange extract
Sage
Pizza sauce
Maple extract
Dill weed
Unflavored gelatin
Pumpkin pie spice
Cheesecake flavor
Sugar-free instant pudding mix
Cocoa powder

With all these food stuffs in your pantry, you definitely have a wide range of options. However, what happens when you have to eat out?

Eating Out While On The Keto Diet

When eating out, be aware that even naturally Keto foods are likely to be processed or contain high carb sauces and other addictives. For this reason, get to know details on how foods served in restaurants are prepared and the type of sauces and condiments used.

It is always better to opt for a salad and condiments like olive oil that are unlikely to have additives. Also, you are better off taking a glass of water of a glass of wine rather than juice.

Chapter 5: 21-Day Diet Meal Plan

<u>Week 1</u>

Day 1

Breakfast
Bacon Spinach Egg Cup

Lunch
Creamy Lobster

Dinner
Nacho Chicken Casserole

Snack
Skillet Pizza

Dessert
Mock Cinnabon

Day 2

Breakfast
Chorizo Breakfast Casserole

Lunch
Glazed Chicken

Dinner
Zucchini Lasagna

Snack
Stuffed Celery

Dessert
Chocolate Peanut Butter Fudge

Day 3

Breakfast
French Toast Casserole

Lunch
Turkey Meatballs

Dinner
Beef Brisket with Sweet potatoes

Snack
Almond Crackers

Dessert
Strawberry Cheesecake

Day 4

Breakfast
Italian Baked Eggs

Lunch
Chicken Casserole

Dinner
Lunch's leftovers

Snack
Cauliflower popcorn

Day 5

Breakfast
Squash Casserole

Lunch
Creamy Lobster

Dinner
Orange and Sage Glazed Duck Breast

Snack
Skillet Pizza

Dessert
Pumpkin Custard

Day 6

Breakfast
Shakshouka

Lunch
Previous night's leftovers

Dinner
Keto Chili

Snack
Stuffed Celery

Dessert
Baked Cream Cheese

Day 7

Breakfast
Italian Baked Eggs

Lunch
Tangy Pear Salad

Dinner
Spinach Salad

Snack
Nutty Almond Crackers

Dessert
Mock Cinnabon

Week 2

Day 1

Breakfast
Bacon Spinach Egg Cup

Lunch
Spinach Salad

Dinner
Fish Cakes

Snack
Cheese Chips

Dessert
Pumpkin Custard

Day 2

Breakfast
Chorizo Breakfast Casserole

Lunch
Chicken Casserole

Dinner
Nacho Chicken Casserole

Snack
Crispy Baked Radish Chips

Dessert
Baked Cream Cheese

Day 3

Breakfast
French Toast Casserole

Lunch
Seafood Creole

Dinner
Zucchini Lasagna

Snack
Keto Trail Mix

Dessert
Mock Cinnabon

Day 4

Breakfast
Italian Baked Eggs

Lunch
Turkey Meatballs

Dinner
Lunch's leftovers

Snack
Cauliflower popcorn

Dessert
Pumpkin Custard

Day 5

Breakfast
Squash Casserole

Lunch
Creamy Lobster

Dinner
Nacho Chicken Casserole

Snack
Stuffed Celery

Day 6

Breakfast
Shakshouka

Lunch
Seafood Creole

Dinner
Zucchini Lasagna

Snack
Almond Crackers

Dessert
Chocolate Peanut Butter
Fudge

Day 7

Breakfast
Squash Casserole

Lunch
Creamy Lobster

Dinner
Fish cakes

Snack
Cauliflower popcorn

Dessert
Strawberry Cheesecake

Week 3

Day 1

Breakfast
Italian Baked Eggs

Lunch
Glazed Chicken

Dinner
Nacho Chicken Casserole

Snack
Stuffed Celery

Day 2

Breakfast
French Toast Casserole

Lunch
Tangy Pear Salad

Dinner
Zucchini Lasagna

Snack
Almond Crackers

Dessert
Pumpkin Custard

Day 3

Breakfast
Bacon Spinach Egg Cup

Lunch
Chicken Cordon Bleu
Casserole

Dinner
Spinach Salad

Snack
½ avocado seasoned with
pepper and salt

Dessert
Baked Cream Cheese

Day 4

Breakfast
Chorizo Breakfast Casserole

Lunch
Seafood Creole

Dinner
Orange and Sage Glazed Duck
Breast

Snack
Skillet Pizza

Dessert
Mock Cinnabon

Day 5

Breakfast
Italian Baked Eggs

Lunch
Creamy Lobster

Dinner
Keto Chili

Snack
Cheese Chips

Dessert
Pumpkin Custard

Day 6

Breakfast
Squash Casserole

Lunch
Glazed Chicken

Dinner
Spinach Salad

Snack
Crispy Baked Radish Chips

Dessert
Berry smoothie

Day 7

Breakfast
Shakshouka

Lunch
Tangy Pear Salad

Dinner
Beef brisket with sweet potatoes

Snack
Keto Trail Mix

Dessert
Mock Cinnabon

The subsequent chapters will cover the recipes for meals mentioned above.

Chapter 6: Breakfast

Shakshouka

Serves 4

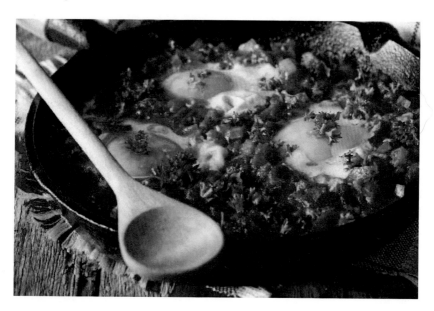

Ingredients

1 cup thinly sliced red bell pepper
1 teaspoon ground cumin
3 tablespoons olive oil
1 1/3 cups chopped onions
1 hot Chile pepper, seeded and finely chopped
1 teaspoon salt
2 cloves garlic, minced, or to taste
2 1/2 cups chopped tomatoes
4 eggs
1 teaspoon paprika

Directions

1. Heat olive oil in a skillet, over medium heat and then stir in bell peppers, garlic and onions.

2. Stir the veggies and cook them for around 5 minutes or until softened and the onion is translucent.

3. Into a bowl, mix together paprika, tomatoes, cumin, Chile pepper and salt. Pour the mixture into the skillet, and stir to incorporate the ingredients.

4. Simmer the mixture while uncovered for about 10 minutes.

5. Into the mixture, make 4 indentations for the eggs and then crack the eggs into them.

6. Let the eggs cook while covered for another 5 minutes. When done, the eggs should be firm but not dry.

Nutritional Information Per Serving: Fat 14g, Protein 7g, Net Carbs 6g

Squash Casserole

Serves 10

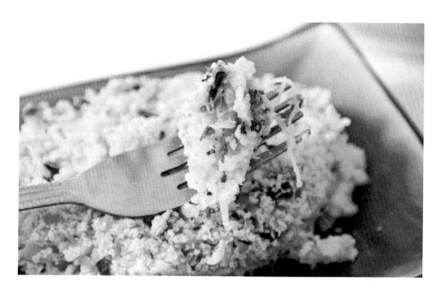

Ingredients

1/2 cup chopped onion
1/4 cup butter, melted
1 cup shredded Cheddar cheese
4 cups sliced yellow squash
35 buttery round crackers, crushed
2 eggs, beaten
3/4 cup milk
1 teaspoon salt
Ground black pepper to taste
2 tablespoons butter

Directions

1. Preheat the oven to 400ºF. Meanwhile, add onion and squash into a large skillet and pour in some water.

2. Cook for about 5 minutes, covered over medium heat. Once the squash is tender, drain the mixture and transfer to a large bowl.

3. Combine together cheese and cracker crumbs in a medium bowl and then stir half of the cracker mixture into the onion mixture.

4. Combine milk and eggs in a small bowl and then add it into the squash-cracker mixture.

5. Stir in the melted butter and season with pepper and salt. Spread the mixture onto a baking dish and then sprinkle with cracker mixture. Dot with 2 tablespoons of butter.

6. Bake for 25 minutes or until lightly browned.

Nutritional Information Per Serving: Fat 11g, Protein 5g, Net Carbs 4g

Italian Baked Eggs

Serves 4

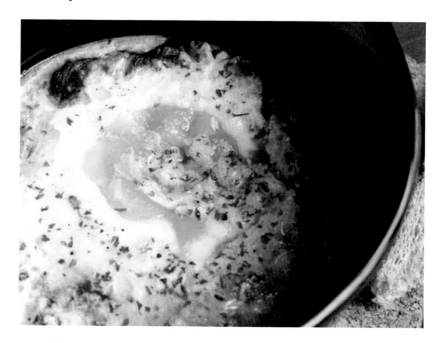

Ingredients

8 tablespoons heavy whipping cream
1/3 cups marinara sauce
4 tablespoons finely shredded cheese
2 teaspoons red pepper flakes
Salt
Freshly ground black pepper
6 teaspoons chopped fresh flat-leaf parsley
8 eggs
8 teaspoons olive oil
8 slices Keto Flax Bread

Directions

1. Preheat your oven to 400° F.

2. Spoon the marinara sauce to about ¼ high into a baking dish. Then sprinkle with parsley, red pepper flakes, black pepper and salt.

3. At the center of the sauce, make a narrow well. Crack in the eggs into a ramekin and pour over the sauce.

4. Sprinkle with the cheese, cream and olive oil and then season with pepper and salt.

5. Bake in the oven for around 10 to 12minutes. To serve, top with toasted low-carb bread.

Nutritional Information Per Serving: Fat 27g, Protein 9g, Net Carbs 5g

French Toast Casserole

Serves 6

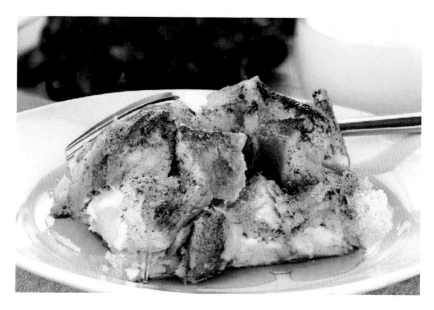

Ingredients

1 1/2 cups milk
4 eggs
1 teaspoon vanilla extract
5 cups cubed Keto bread
1/4 cup splenda
2 teaspoons ground cinnamon

Directions

1. Preheat your oven to 350°F and then use cooking spray to coat a 9x13 baking dish.

2. Use bread cubes to line the bottom of the baking dish

3. Into a bowl, beat in eggs, 1 teaspoon cinnamon, vanilla extract, 2 tablespoons sweetener and milk.

4. Pour this egg mixture into the baking dish that has bread cubes and allow to incorporate for at least 10 minutes. Alternatively, refrigerate overnight.

5. Combine 1 teaspoon cinnamon and 2 tablespoons sweetener and sprinkle it over the casserole.

6. Bake the contents in the oven for about 30-40 minutes. Remove from oven after the casserole is set and the topping is crunchy.

Nutritional Information Per Serving: Fat 3g, Protein 5g, Net Carbs 3g

Chorizo Breakfast Casserole

Serves 6

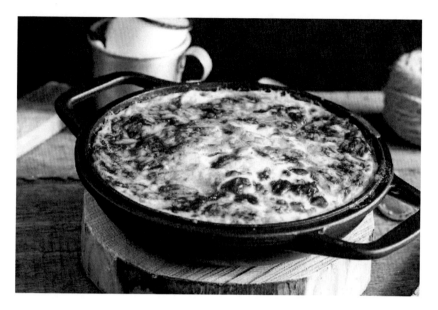

Ingredients

1/2 yellow onion, diced
1 teaspoon garlic powder
1 teaspoon salt
1 teaspoon onion powder
1 sweet potato, shredded
12 eggs, whisked
1 lb. chorizo, cooked and diced
2 tablespoons hot sauces
1 teaspoon pepper

Directions

1. Heat a skillet and then add chorizo. Allow to cook until it starts to crumble.

2. As the chorizo cooks, shred the sweet potato and dice the onion.

3. Beat the eggs in a bowl and then add the onion, cooked meat and sweet potato. Then add the other ingredients and combine well.

4. Grease a glass dish and add the egg-meat mixture. Cook until the eggs aren't runny; for about 15-30 minutes.

5. Allow to sit for 10 minutes before serving.

Nutritional Information Per Serving: Fat 18g, Protein 12g, Net Carbs 5g

Bacon Spinach Egg Cup

Serves 6

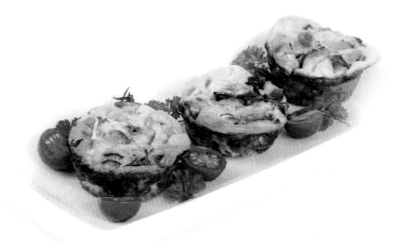

Ingredients

6 eggs
2 slices onions, chopped
4 mushrooms, chopped
1 1/4 cups shredded Colby-jack cheese, divided
1 pinch salt and ground black pepper
1 pinch onion powder
1/2 (12-ounce) package frozen chopped spinach
1 tablespoon heavy whipping cream
4 slices thick-cut bacon, diced
1/4 green bell pepper, chopped
1/2 teaspoon salt
1/4 teaspoon ground black pepper
1 pinch garlic powder

Directions

1. Preheat your oven to 350ºF and then use cooking spray to coat 12 muffin cups.

2. Over medium-high heat, cook and stir bacon in a skillet until crisp for around 10 minutes.

3. Put the bacon to a separate bowl but reserve the bacon grease in the skillet.

4. In the skillet that has reserved grease, combine onion, green bell pepper, salt, spinach, ground pepper and mushrooms.

5. Cook the mixture for about 5 minutes to soften then transfer this mixture into a separate bowl. Refrigerate for around 5 minutes.

6. Into a bowl, whisk together cream and eggs and then stir 1 cup Jack cheese, onion powder, ¼ teaspoon ground pepper, garlic powder and ½ teaspoon salt.

7. Remove the veggies from the freezer and add into the to the egg mixture alongside the bacon. Mix gently to incorporate.

8. Into each muffin cup, scoop ¼ cup of the egg mixture and then top each using the remaining cheese.

9. Now bake for around 20 minutes until the egg cups are set.

Nutritional Information Per Serving: Fat 6g, Protein 8g, Net Carbs 2g

Chapter 7: Lunch

Fish Cakes

Serves 4

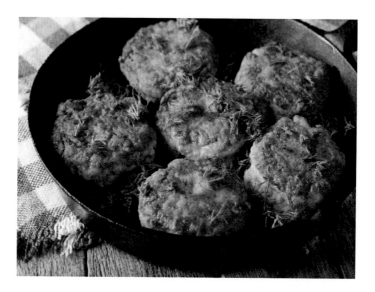

Ingredients

6 basil leaves
6 ounces fresh shrimp, drained
1 tablespoon Italian seasoning
1/2 cup Keto bread crumbs
1 bunch fresh parsley
1 egg
6 oz. fresh bay scallops
5 sun-dried tomatoes, chopped
4 tablespoons almond flour
4 tablespoons olive oil, divided
1/2 medium onion
4 cloves garlic
2 fresh hot Chile peppers, seeded
1 (9-ounce) can tuna, drained

Directions

1. Heat a tablespoon of olive oil in a skillet, over medium heat and then stir in scallops.

2. Cook the mixture until white on all sides. Drain and then set aside the scallops.

3. Put garlic, egg, 1 tablespoon olive oil, sundried tomatoes and onion into a food processor,

4. Then add in Italian seasoning, basil leaves, parsley and chilies and pulse on medium setting to obtain a chopped consistency.

5. Now add in tuna, shrimp and scallops and pulse on low. Pour in breadcrumbs and continue to pulse to obtain a firm and sticky puree.

6. Form the puree into palm-size patties that measure 1 inch thick and set onto a plate. Cover and keep it chilled for 1 hour.

7. Heat 2 tablespoons olive oil in a large skillet, over medium. Then dust the patties lightly in flour as you shake off any excess.

8. Put the patties into the skillet and cook on both sides until golden brown.

Nutritional Information Per Serving: Fat 24g, Protein 24g, Net Carbs 9g

Glazed Chicken

Serves 4

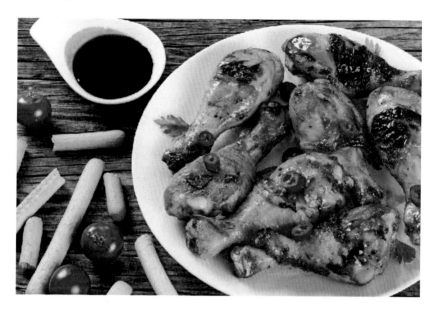

Ingredients

1 cup water
1/2 cup balsamic vinegar
1 peeled and bruised garlic clove
8 chicken drumsticks , skin on
2 tablespoons of sweetener
1 hot chili pepper, slit open and seeds removed
1/3 cup soy sauce

Directions

1. Place all the ingredients into a saucepan, and then bring to a boil over high heat.

2. Lower the heat and allow to simmer for 20 minutes. Remember to remove scum that may rise to the surface.

3. Gently increase the heat as you turn drumsticks regularly in the liquid. Continue to cook until the liquid reduces.

4. Arrange the chicken on a serving platter and then remove chili and garlic clove from the liquid.

5. Now spoon the glaze over and serve.

Nutritional Information Per Serving: Fat 3g, Protein 10g, Net Carbs 8g

Creamy Lobster

Serves 4

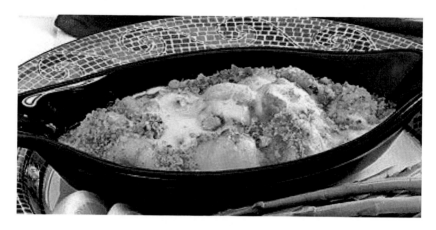

Ingredients

2 tablespoons dry sherry

1 pinch cayenne pepper

2 eggs yolks, beaten

1/2 cup heavy cream

1/4 cup butter

1 pinch ground nutmeg

3/4 lb. cooked lobster, broken into chunks

1/2 teaspoon salt

Directions

1. Whisk together heavy cream and egg yolks in a small bowl until well incorporated and then set it aside.

2. Melt butter in a saucepan over medium heat, and then stir in the sherry and egg yolk mixture.

3. Cook the ingredients stirring throughout until the mixture thickens. Ensure that it doesn't boil.

4. Once ready, remove from heat and season with cayenne, nutmeg and salt. Then add lobster and then return to the pan.

5. Cook gently over low-heat until heated through and then serve with some steamed vegetables.

Nutritional Information Per Serving: Fat 16g, Protein 28g, Net Carbs 8g

Seafood Creole

Serves 6

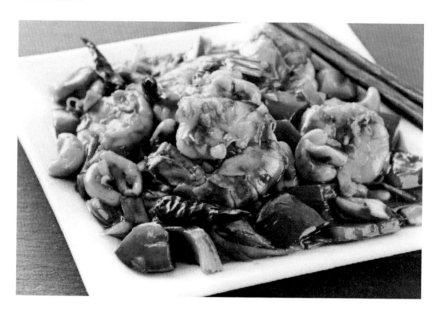

Ingredients

1 1/4 cups chicken stock
3/4 cup chopped green bell pepper
1/2 teaspoon dried sweet basil
1 cup peeled chopped tomato
1/2 teaspoon cayenne pepper
1 cup canned tomato sauce
1 1/2 teaspoons garlic cloves, minced
3/4 cup chopped celery
1 lb. haddock fillets cut into pieces
1/4 cup butter
1 lb. bay scallops
1 lb. peeled and deveined shrimp
3/4 teaspoon dried oregano
1/2 teaspoon salt
1/2 teaspoon ground white pepper

1/2 teaspoon ground black pepper
1/2 teaspoon dried thyme leaves
3/4 cup chopped onion
1/2 teaspoon hot pepper sauce, cholula
2 bay leaves

Directions

1. In a small bowl, mix cayenne pepper, white pepper, salt, oregano, basil and thyme and set aside.

2. Melt butter in a large Dutch oven, over medium heat and then stir in celery, onion, tomato, garlic and bell pepper.

3. Cook the mixture for about 5 minutes or until translucent. Then stir in hot pepper sauce, chicken stock, bay leaves and tomato sauce.

4. Now lower the heat and let it simmer for some time. Stir in seasoning, mix and continue to simmer for around 20 minutes for the flavors to blend.

5. Finally stir in haddock, shrimp and bay scallops and then bring the sauce to a simmer. Serve.

Nutritional Information Per Serving: Fat 9g, Protein 30g, Net Carbs 6g

Chicken Cordon Bleu Casserole

Serves 6

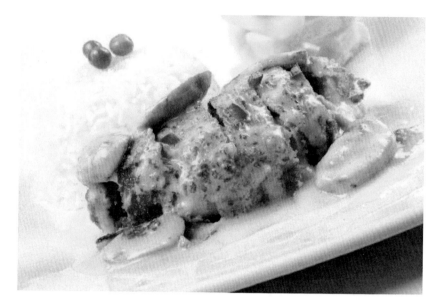

Ingredients

Dry keto crumbs
1/2 cup milk
1 egg, mixed with the milk
8 ounces ham, diced
1 (10 3/4 ounce) can cream of chicken soup
1 cup milk
2 lbs. skinless chicken breasts
8 ounces Swiss cheese, cubed

Directions

1. Preheat your oven to 350°F.

2. Dip the chicken into milk and egg mixture. Toss the ingredients with bread crumbs then add in little oil until turn golden.

3. Place the chicken into a baking dish, and then add ham and cheese.

4. Mix soup with 1 cup of milk to cover up the chicken.

5. Bake in the preheated oven until tender and bubbly. This should take 30-35 minutes.

Nutritional Information Per Serving: Fat 3g, Protein 18g, Net Carbs 4g

Turkey Meatballs

Serves 5

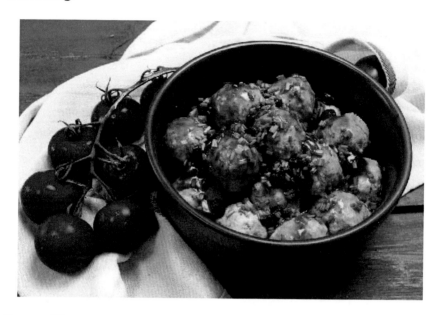

Ingredients

2 large handful spinach
1/2 teaspoon salt
2 large eggs
3 small red chili peppers
1 oz. pork sausage rinds
1 small onion
10 slices bacon
2 lbs. ground turkey
1/2 medium green pepper
1/2 teaspoon pepper
3 sprigs thyme

Directions

1. Preheat the oven to 400ºF and then use foil to line a baking sheet and then add in the bacon.

2. Now put the bacon in the preheated oven and cook until crisp, in about 30 minutes. Remove from the oven and set aside. Drain off the fat into a bowl.

3. Meanwhile, dice and add other ingredients into a food processor apart from the bacon and turkey. Add the processed ingredients to the ground turkey and mix completely.

4. Make 20 meatballs and lay them on the same sheet that had the cooked bacon.

5. Cook the meatballs until the juices run clear, for around 15-20 minutes. To

each meatball, skewer 2-3 pieces of the bacon.

Nutritional Information Per Serving: Fat 9g, Protein 7g, Net Carbs 4g

Chapter 8: Dinner

Zucchini Lasagna

Serves 6

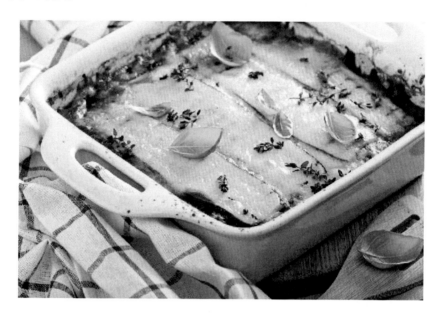

Ingredients

1/4 teaspoon ground nutmeg
1/2 cup mozzarella cheese
12 oz. button mushrooms
1 teaspoon dried oregano
1 1/2 cups diced onions
3 large zucchini
1 tablespoon salt
Cooking spray
2 minced garlic cloves
3 cups chopped tomatoes
3-4 cups raw spinach leaves
1 tablespoon dried basil
1/4 teaspoon black pepper

Directions

1. Slice the zucchini into 1/8-inch strips in a bowl and then season with salt. Toss to coat the strips and then lay them on paper towels. Set aside for about 1 hour.

2. Using a non-stick spray, coat a large saucepan and then set it over medium heat. Add the onion and cook for about 2 minutes or until softened.

3. Add in garlic and cook for 20 seconds then follow with mushrooms. Cook for about 7 minutes, until the mushroom reduces to a glaze.

4. At this point, stir in nutmeg, oregano, basil, tomatoes and pepper. Cook the mixture for about 25 minutes. By now the tomato should start to break down and the sauce thicken.

5. Position the rack in the center of the oven, and preheat to 350°F.

6. Use paper towels to blot moisture from zucchini strips and then lay a third of the strips lengthwise into a 9x13-inch baking dish. Lay them like lasagna noodles and then top with a third of the sauce and third of shredded cheese.

7. Now put half of the zucchini strips on top and top with half the remaining sauce and cheese.

8. Repeat with the remaining zucchini strips, sauce and cheese and then bake uncovered for 45 minutes.

9. Once it starts bubbling, allow to cool for 10 minutes and then serve.

Nutritional Information Per Serving: Fat 4g, Protein 8g, Net Carbs 7g

Nacho Chicken Casserole

Serves 6

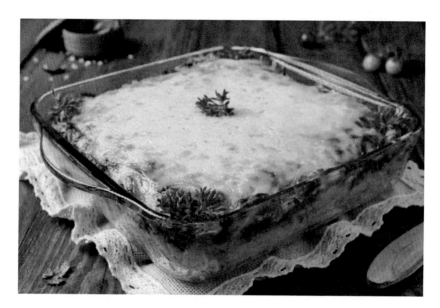

Ingredients

4 oz. Cheddar cheese
1 cup green chilies and tomato
1 medium jalapeno pepper
1/4 cup sour cream
1.75 lbs. chicken thighs, boneless skinless
1 1/2 teaspoons chili seasoning
2 tablespoons olive oil
3 tablespoons parmesan cheese
1 packet frozen cauliflower
Salt and pepper to taste
4 oz. cream cheese

Directions

1. Preheat the oven to 375° F. Meanwhile, chop and season the chicken and then cook until browned in olive oil over medium heat.

2. Into a bowl, add in sour cream, cream cheese and ¾ of the cheddar and then stir together until mixed together.

3. Add in green chili and the tomatoes and mix well, and then transfer the ingredients to a casserole dish.

4. Microwave frozen cauliflower until it's done then blend it together with the remaining cheese using an immersion blender. Process into mashed potato-like consistency.

5. Season the cauliflower. Then cut jalapeno pepper into chunks.

6. Spread the cauliflower over the casserole and sprinkle with jalapeno.

7.Bake the casserole for 15-20 minutes and then serve.

Nutritional Information Per Serving: Fat 17g, Protein 7g, Net Carbs 5g

Beef Brisket

Serves 8

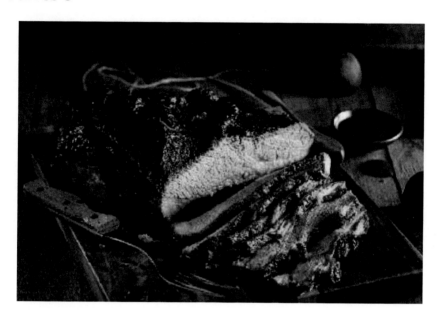

Ingredients

2 cloves garlic, minced
2 tablespoons tapioca
½ cup salsa
½ cup hoision sauce
3 ½ lbs. beef brisket, trimmed
2lbs. sweet potatoes, peeled and cut

Directions

1. Place the sweet potatoes in a 6-quart slow cooker.

2. Put the beef brisket on top then combine garlic, tapioca, salsa and hoisin sauce. Pour this sauce mixture over the beef, cover and cook for 10 hurs on low heat and for 5 hours on high heat setting.

3. Transfer themeat to a cutting board and cut into slices across the grain.

4. Serve the potatoes over the beef.

Nutritional Information Per Serving: Fat 42g, Protein 44g, Net Carbs 9g

Spinach Salad

Serves 4

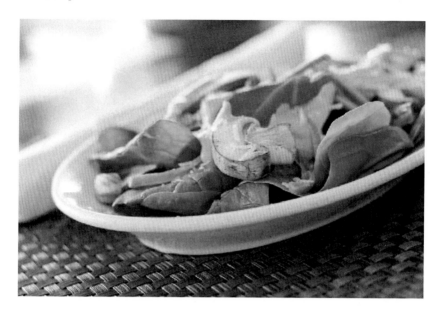

Ingredients

1/2 cup vegetable oil
1/4 teaspoon ground black pepper
1/2 teaspoon celery seed
1/2 teaspoon salt
1/2 onion, chopped
3 eggs
1/4 lb. bacon
1 lb. spinach, rinsed and chopped
1 1/3 ounces croutons (Keto bread)
2 tablespoons sliced fresh mushrooms
2 1/2 tablespoons cider vinegar
1 1/2 teaspoons Dijon Mustard
5 sachets Splenda

Directions

1. Put eggs into a saucepan and then add in cold water to completely cover the eggs. Bring the contents to a boil.

2. Cover and remove the eggs from heat then let it stand in hot water for about 10 minutes.

3. Remove from water, cool for a few minutes and then peel and chop them.

4. Place the bacon in a large and deep skillet, and then cook it over high heat until browned evenly. Drain the bacon, crumble and set it aside.

5. Now make the dressing by mixing vinegar, Splenda, onion, pepper, salt, Dijon Mustard and celery seed in a blender. Process until smooth.

6. In a large salad bowl, mix together bacon, mushrooms, croutons and eggs then toss evenly.

7. Drizzle the dressing over the salad to lightly coat, toss and then serve.

Nutritional Information Per Serving: Fat 22g, Protein 9g, Net Carbs 8g

Keto Chili

Serves 8

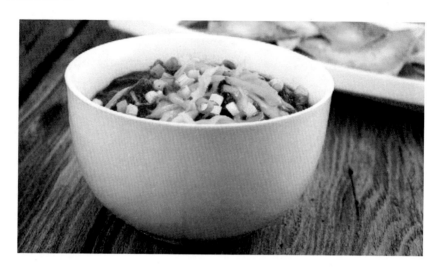

Ingredients

1 lb. hot Italian sausage
1 can tomato sauce
1 large green pepper
2 tablespoons curry powder
1 teaspoon onion powder
2 tablespoons cumin
1 lb. ground beef
1 large yellow pepper
1 medium white onion
2 tablespoons chili powder
1 tablespoon butter
1 teaspoon salt
1 teaspoon freshly ground black pepper
1 tablespoon minced garlic
1 tablespoon organic coconut oil

Directions

1. Add butter and coconut oil to a pan over medium heat, and heat until melted. Then add onions, pepper and garlic. Sauté until done.

2. Over medium heat, warm a pot then add ground beef and sausage. Cook the meat until browned and then add pepper and salt to taste.

3. Into the pot, add onion powder, tomato sauce, peppers, garlic, onion and chili powder.

4. Cook the meat and spices for 20 minutes then add in cumin and curry powder. Cook for 10 additional minutes while stirring often.

5. Allow to simmer for up to 2 hours to incorporate the flavor.

Nutritional Information Per Serving: Fat 22g, Protein 10g Net Carbs 3g

Orange and Sage Glazed Duck Breast

Serves 4

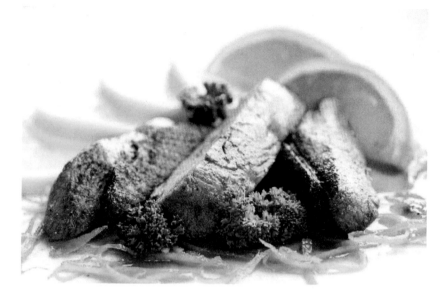

Ingredients

3 tablespoons swerve
3 tablespoons heavy cream
3 cups spinach
6 tablespoons butter
3 (6 oz.) duck breasts
1 1/2 teaspoons orange extract
3/4 teaspoon sage

Directions

1. First score the duck skin on top of the duck breast and then season with pepper and salt.

2. Add butter into a pan over medium-low heat and then lower the heat for the butter to lightly brown.

3. Once browned, add orange extract and sage and continue cooking until the butter is deep amber colored.

4. Into a separate pan, put the breast and then heat over medium high for few minutes. Flip the meat occasionally until crispy.

5. Now add heavy cream to the mixture and stir to incorporate. Pour the cream sage butter mixture onto the duck breast and allow to coat.

6. Cook the breast for a few more minutes before serving. If desired, you can wilt some spinach in the pan to prepare a sauce.

Nutritional Information Per Serving: Fat 6g, Protein 24g, Net Carbs 0g

Chapter 9: Snacks

Cauliflower Popcorn

Serves 4

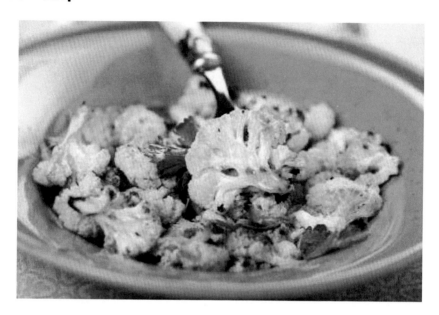

Ingredients

1 teaspoon salt, to taste
4 tablespoons olive oil
1 head cauliflower

Directions

1. Preheat oven to 425 degrees.

2. Trim the cauliflower and discard the core and thick stems and then cut the florets into pieces.

3. Combine the salt and olive oil in a bowl and then add in the cauliflower pieces and toss to coat.

4. Use parchment paper to line a baking sheet and then spread the cauliflower pieces on the baking sheet.

5. Roast for 1 hour or until golden brown making sure to turn 3 or 4 times.

Nutritional Information Per Serving: Fat 1g, Protein 2g, Net Carbs 3g

Almond Crackers

Serves 5

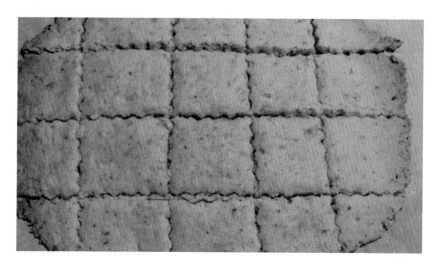

Ingredients

1/2 teaspoon salt
2 tablespoons finely chopped walnuts
2 tablespoons water
1 cup almond flour
1 1/2 teaspoons flax seed meal
1 1/2 teaspoons olive oil

Directions

1. Preheat your oven to 350ºF and then line baking sheets using parchment paper.

2. Mix flaxseed meal, walnuts, almond flour and salt in a bowl, until fully combined.

3. Then add in olive oil and water and mix until the dough is moist and is held together.

4.Once done, turn the dough on the baking sheet and then cover using another parchment paper.

5. Using a rolling pin, roll the dough into a 1 by 16-inch thick rectangle. Remove the parchment cover and cut the slices of dough to make an even rectangle.

6. Add the excess dough to the end of rectangle or its corners then re-roll to achieve uniform thickness.

7. Now use a pizza cutter to cut the dough into 1-inch squares, then bake in the oven for about 15 minutes.

8. Once the outside edges of the dough are browned, cool the crackers and break it into squares. If desired, serve with salsa and guacamole.

Nutritional Information Per Serving: Fat 26g, Protein 3g, Net Carbs 5g

Stuffed Celery

Serves 4

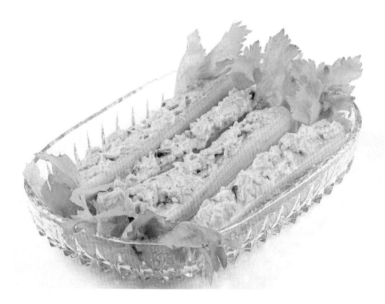

Ingredients

1 dash onion powder
1 1/2 teaspoons dried parsley flakes
1/4 teaspoon dried thyme
8 celery ribs, 3 inch long
1 (8-ounce) package cream cheese
1/3 cup carrot, shredded

Directions

1. Combine carrot, cream cheese and seasoning in a small bowl.

2. Then use the cream mixture to fill each celery piece.

3. Cover and keep refrigerated for 1-2 hours.

Nutritional Information Per Serving: Fat 8g, Protein 1g, Net Carbs 3g

Skillet Pizza

Serves 2

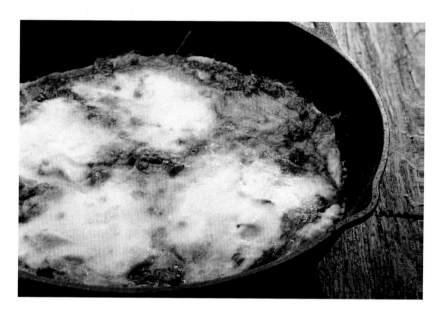

Ingredients

2 mushrooms, sliced
2 tablespoons 1 -2 turkey pepperoni, chopped
4 tablespoons mozzarella cheese
2 tablespoons pizza sauce
4 slices deli ham
Dash oregano

Directions

1. Preheat a non-stick skillet. Then lightly brown ham slices on each side.

2. Over the browned ham, spread the pizza sauce and add the toppings; followed by shredded cheese on top. Sprinkle the mixture with oregano.

3. Cover and cook gently on medium low heat, for about 1-2minutes.

Nutritional Information Per Serving: Fat 7g, Protein 11g, Net Carbs 5g

Keto Trail Mix

Serves 4

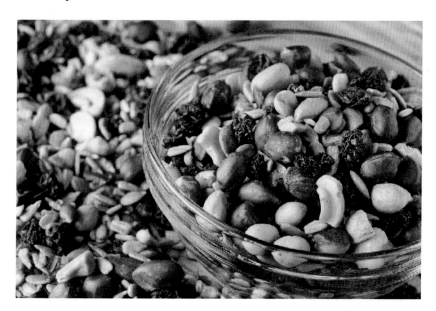

Ingredients

1/2 cup raisins
1 cup sunflower seeds
1/2 cup shredded coconut, unsweetened
1 cup almonds

Directions

1. Combine all ingredients in a bowl.

2. Serve and enjoy.

Nutritional Information Per Serving: Fat 12g, Protein 8g, Net Carbs 10g

Baked Radish Chips

Serves 4

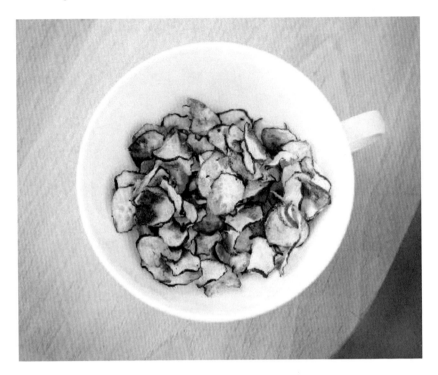

Ingredients

10 -15 large radishes
Salt and pepper, to taste

Directions

1. Preheat the oven to 375°F and coat a cookie sheet with non-stick spray.

2. Slice the radishes into thin chips and spread the chips onto the prepared cookie sheet.

3. Use cooking spray to lightly mist radish slices and then season with salt and pepper.

4. Now bake each side for 10 minutes or until crisp.

Nutritional Information Per Serving: Fat 0g, Protein 0g, Net Carbs 5g

Cheese Chips

Serves 2

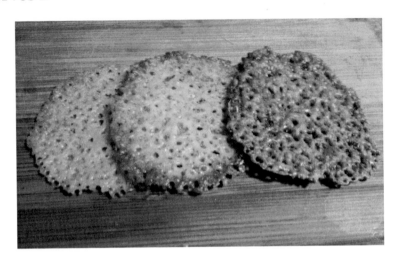

Ingredients

1/4 tablespoon flaxseed meal
1/8 cup Cheddar cheese shredded

Directions

1. Preheat your oven to 425°F.

2. Onto a silicon non-stick pad, make 2 tablespoon moulds of cheese and then spread out some flaxseed on each chip.

3. Once distributed evenly, add the desired seasonings to each chip.

4. Now bake the chips until done and then remove from the oven. Allow to cool and then set onto a plate. Top with low-carb salsa if desired.

Nutritional Information Per Serving: Fat 3g, Protein 2g, Net Carbs 0g

Chapter 10: Desserts

Mock Cinnabon

Serves 4

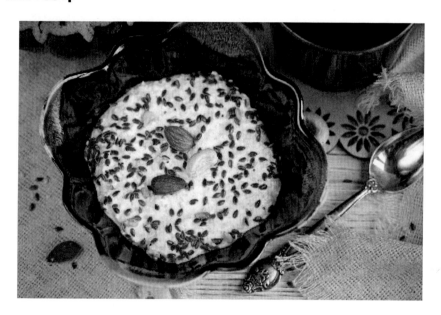

Ingredients

28 pecans halves, toasted
4 packets splenda
2 cups cottage cheese
4 drops maple extract
Ground cinnamon

Directions

1. Combine maple extract, cottage cheese and the Splenda then sprinkle with cinnamon.

2. Top the dessert with pecan halves.

Nutritional Information Per Serving: Fat 2g, Protein 12g, Net Carbs 5g

Baked Cream Cheese

Serves 8

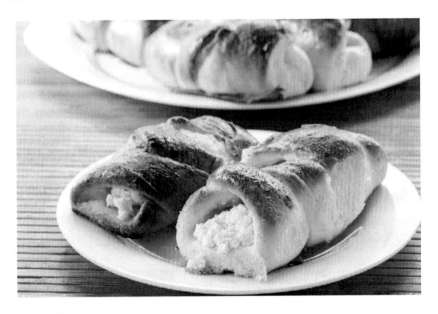

Ingredients

1/2 teaspoon dried dill weed
1 egg yolk, beaten
1/2 (8-ounce) package refrigerated crescent roll
1 (8-ounce) package cream cheese

Directions

1. Preheat your oven to 350°F.

2. Unroll the dough on a lightly floured surface, and then press together the seams to form 12x4 inch rectangle.

3. Use half of the dill to sprinkle one side of the cream cheese. In the center of the dough, place brick of cream cheese dill side down and sprinkle dill on top of cream cheese.

4. Now bring the sides of the dough together to enclose the cream cheese and then press the edges to seal it.

5. Put the dough onto a lightly greased cookie sheet and then brush with a beaten egg.

6. Bake for about 15-18 minutes. Serve warm.

Nutritional Information Per Serving: Fat 13g, Protein 3g, Net Carbs 9g

Pumpkin Custard

Serves 6

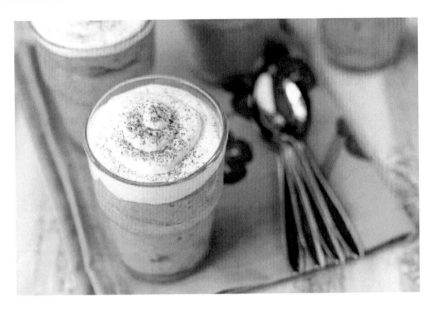

Ingredients

1 12 ounce can evaporated milk
6 gingersnaps
2 beaten eggs
ground nutmeg
4 teaspoons cornstarch
1 15 ounce can pumpkin
1 envelope unflavored gelatin
3/4 teaspoon pumpkin pie spice
1/8 teaspoon salt
14 packets splenda
frozen whipped topping, thawed

Directions

1. Combine salt, cornstarch, gelatin and pumpkin pie spice into a large sauce pan.

2. Then stir in evaporated milk and pumpkin and allow to stand for 5 minutes to soften gelatin.

3. Over medium heat, cook and stir for about 2 minutes until the mixture bubbles.

4. Then remove from heat and stir in 1 cup hot mixture into the eggs. Return the egg mixture into the saucepan.

5. Cook custard for 2 minutes over low heat, stirring regularly. Then remove from heat and stir in favorite sweetener.

6. Into the bottom of six 6-ounce custard cups, put a gingersnap and then spoon the pumpkin mixture into the cups.

7. Cover and keep into the fridge for 6-24 hours. To serve, sprinkle with nutmeg and then garnish with whipped topping.

Strawberry Cheesecake

Serves 12

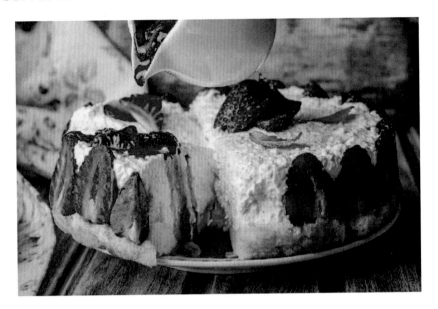

Ingredients

1 1/2 cups milk

1/4 teaspoon ground nutmeg

1/4 teaspoon ground cinnamon

2 pints fresh strawberries, sliced

1 (1-ounce) package cheesecake flavor sugar-free instant pudding mix

3 tablespoons butter, melted

3/4 cup keto graham cracker crumbs

1 (8-ounce) package cream cheese, softened

Directions

1. Mix together melted butter, nutmeg, cracker crumbs and cinnamon in a bowl.

2. Press the mixture into an 8-inch pie dish, and then refrigerate as you prepare the filling.

3. Beat cream cheese in a mixing bowl with an electric mixer, on medium speed.

4. Set the speed to low and then gradually beat in milk. Scrap the cream cheese using rubber spatula from sides of the bowl.

5. Now beat in pudding mix to obtain a thick and smooth paste.

6. At the bottom of the graham cracker crust, spoon half of the cream cheese and spread half of the berries over the filling.

7. Make another cheesecake layer and strawberry layer then cool for at least 1 hour. Serve it once set and cold.

Nutritional Information Per Serving: Fat 11g, Protein 3g, Net Carbs 10g

Chocolate Peanut Butter Fudge

Serves 32

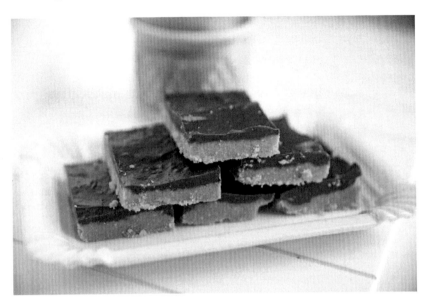

Ingredients

1/4 cup cocoa powder
1/2 cup splenda granular
1/2 teaspoon vanilla
8 ounces cream cheese
1 cup butter
1 cup peanut butter

Directions

1.Into a microwave-safe bowl, add butter, peanut butter and cream cheese and then microwave to melt the butter and whisk the ingredients.

2. Then add in splenda, cocoa powder and vanilla and whisk to obtain smooth consistency.

3. Pour the batter into an 8x8 pan lined with foil and keep in the refrigerator until set.

Conclusion

I hope you have learned about the Ketogenic diet and are excited to get started with it.

Thank you and all the best with your new lean self!

15116063R00052

Made in the USA
Lexington, KY
11 November 2018